COMPLETE GUIDE TO ENDOMETRIAL ABLATION

Essential Manual To Minimally Invasive Treatment For Heavy Menstrual Bleeding, Uterine Health, And Long Term Relief

DR. BRUNO HORAN

Copyright © 2023 by Dr. Bruno Horan

All rights reserved. Except for brief quotations embodied in critical reviews and certain other noncommercial uses permitted by copyright law, no part of this publication may be reproduced, distributed, or transmitted in any form or by any means, Including photocopying, recording, or other electronic or mechanical methods, without the prior written permission of the publisher.

Disclaimer:

The information provided in this book, is intended for general informational purposes only and should not be considered as professional advice.

The author has made every effort to ensure the accuracy of the information presented. However, readers are advised to consult with a qualified healthcare professional before attempting any herbal remedies or making significant changes to their wellness routine. Individual health conditions vary, and what may be suitable for one person may not be appropriate for another.

It is important to note that the author is not in any endorsement deal, partnership, or affiliation with any organization, brand, or company mentioned in this book. Any references to specific products or services are based on the author's personal experience or general knowledge and do not imply an endorsement or promotion of those products or services

Contents

CHAPTER ONE 15
  ANATOMY AND PHYSIOLOGY OF THE UTERUS 15
    The Uterus's Structure 16
    The Endometrium's Function In The Menstrual Cycle 18
    Control Of Hormones 19
    Typical Uterine Conditions 20
    Imaging Methods And Diagnostic Instruments 22

CHAPTER TWO 25
  CONTRAINDICATIONS AND INDICATIONS 25
    The Cause Of Excessive Menstrual Bleeding 26
    Polyps, Fibroids, And Additional Growths 27
    Knowing What Endometrial Hyperplasia Is 28
    Who Must Steer Clear Of Endometrial Ablation? .. 29
    Essential Pre-procedure Examinations 30

CHAPTER THREE 33
  ENDOMETRIAL ABLATION PROCEDURE TYPES 33
    Ablation Of Thermal Balloons 33
    Ablation Using Radiofrequency 34
    Ablation Via Hydrothermal Process 35

   Ablation Of Microwaves 36
CHAPTER FOUR 39
  BEFORE THE PROCEDURE....................................39
   Preliminary Medical Assessment 39
   Pre-Procedure Drugs And Their Applications.......40
   Dietary Guidelines And Restrictions....................40
   Getting Ready For Procedure Day......................41
   Emotional And Psychological Readiness 41
CHAPTER FIVE 43
  DAY OF THE PROCEDURE 43
   Process Of Arrival And Check-In 43
   Options For Anesthesia And Their Impacts.........44
   Overview Of The Process Step-By-Step..............45
   Length And Experience In The Rehab Room.......46
   Quick Postoperative Care 46
CHAPTER SIX...49
  RESTORATION AFTER PROCEDURE 49
   Normal Timetable For Recuperation...................50
   Handling Soreness And Unease 52
   Activity Limitations And Suggestions..................53

- Indications Of Complications And When To Consult A Physician 54
- Recheck Schedules And Extended-Term Care 55

CHAPTER SEVEN 59
OVERSIGHTING GOALS AND RESULTS 59
- Anticipated Shifts In The Menstrual Cycle 60
- Possible Issues And How To Handle Them 61
- Benefits Over Time And Success Rates 62
- Effects On Pregnancy And Fertility 63
- Case Studies And Patient Testimonials 63

CHAPTER EIGHT 65
COMMON QUESTIONS AND ANSWERS 65
- Tips For Comfort And Pain Management 67
- Recuperation Period And Resume Of Regular Activities 68
- Expense, Coverage, And Grant Support 71
- Following Ablation, Long-Term Health And Wellness 72

ABOUT THE BOOK

In the realm of gynecological health, "Endometrial Ablation" emerges as a crucial resource, providing a thorough overview of a surgery that significantly affects women's quality of life. The goal of endometrial ablation is explained in detail in the first section of the book, along with its applicability in treating uterine problems and heavy monthly flow. It charts the development of the process, emphasizing significant turning points and technical breakthroughs that have improved the procedure's effectiveness throughout time.

An examination of the uterus, including its structure, the endometrium's critical function in the monthly cycle, and the hormonal processes that control it, is the basis of the book. By exploring common uterine illnesses and diagnostic resources, the book equips medical professionals and patients with the knowledge they need to make well-informed decisions.

The book's thorough analysis of numerous endometrial ablation techniques is one of its strongest points. Every technique is examined, from radiofrequency to thermal balloon, providing details on the advantages, dangers, and subtleties of each process. Pre-procedure testing, prescription drugs, and dietary recommendations are all covered in detail during the preparation phase, which makes sure patients are well-informed and ready for their trip.

The book acts as a comforting guide for patients on the day of the treatment, helping them through arrival, anesthetic selections, and a detailed rundown of the entire process. It remains a helpful ally even after the procedure, including information on recovery schedules, pain control techniques, and possible side effects to be aware of, along with practical guidance on when to seek medical attention.

The book discusses long-term issues that go beyond the short-term healing phase, such as anticipated alterations in menstrual cycles, consequences for fertility, and the overall effect on health and wellness. Testimonials from patients and case studies add a human touch to the process and provide firsthand knowledge of the life-changing potential of endometrial ablation.

"Endometrial Ablation" is a source of empowerment for women negotiating difficult health-related decisions, not just a clinical guidebook. Its all-encompassing strategy, which combines medical knowledge with kind advice, guarantees that readers will have the information and self-assurance they need to start along the road to a higher standard of living.

A Brief Overview of Endometrial Ablation

The endometrial lining of the uterus is removed or destroyed during endometrial ablation, a medical surgery intended to address irregular uterine bleeding. Menstrual bleeding is caused by this lining. The goal of the surgery is to minimize or completely stop menstrual flow by destroying or ablating it. For women who have heavy periods that interfere with their daily lives and cause anemia, exhaustion, or other issues, it is a good solution.

Endometrial ablation: What is it?

The purpose of endometrial ablation is to reduce or completely stop monthly bleeding, and this is accomplished using a variety of treatments. A doctor puts devices into the uterus through the cervix during the surgery. These devices use radiation, heat, cold, microwave, or radiofrequency energy to kill endometrial tissue. During each menstrual cycle, the tissue in the uterus thickens and sheds.

The procedure's evolution and history

The notion of endometrial ablation has been around for a few decades, progressing from the initial surgical approaches to the current, less intrusive treatments. During the initial treatments, the endometrial lining was surgically removed. Technology and medical knowledge have progressed over time, resulting in the creation of less intrusive and faster-recovery treatments.

Who Needs to Take This Procedure Into Account?

Women who experience severe menstrual bleeding that does not improve with other therapies, such as medication, may want to think about having their endometrium ablation. It is not advised for people who want to keep their fertility intact because the process drastically lowers the likelihood of becoming pregnant. Women with uterine diseases like cancer, recent pregnancies, or specific structural problems might also not be good candidates.

Summary of Various Methods

Endometrial ablation can be performed using a variety of procedures, each with pros and downsides of their own:

Radiofrequency Ablation: This technique heats and destroys endometrial tissue using radiofrequency energy.

The endometrial tissue is frozen during a cryoablation procedure.

Microwave Ablation: Heat is produced and the endometrial lining is destroyed using microwave energy.

Hydrothermal Ablation: This technique ablates the endometrial tissue by heating saline fluid.

Electrosurgical Ablation: This method involves removing the uterine lining using an electric current.

The size and form of the uterus, the patient's medical history, the doctor's preference, and experience all play a role in the procedure selection.

Benefits and Risks

Endometrial ablation is a medical procedure that has advantages and disadvantages. A better quality of life, a major reduction in monthly bleeding or perhaps the full cessation of periods, and the avoidance of more invasive surgeries like hysterectomy are some possible advantages. Infection, harm to the uterus or its surrounding organs, and, less frequently, issues from anesthesia or fluid overload are among the possible risks.

CHAPTER ONE

ANATOMY AND PHYSIOLOGY OF THE UTERUS

A key component of the female reproductive system, the uterus is essential to menstruation, pregnancy, and childbirth. When not expanded by pregnancy, it is about the size and shape of a pear and is located in the pelvic cavity. The uterus is made up of multiple layers: the endometrium, which is the inner lining of the uterus that changes cyclically in response to hormone fluctuations; the myometrium, which is a thick layer of smooth muscle responsible for the uterus's contractions during childbirth; and the outermost layer, known as the serosa, which is a thin layer of tissue covering the uterus.

The corpus, or body of the uterus, is where the fertilized egg implants and matures during pregnancy, and the cervix, which connects the uterus to the vagina and permits the passage of menstrual blood and sperm, are the two main sections of the uterus. The uterus is carefully supported by blood arteries, nerves, and lymphatic systems, which guarantee its role in reproduction.

Comprehending the structure of the uterus is essential for identifying and managing a range of gynecological ailments, such as irregular bleeding, fibroids, and endometrial problems. Healthcare professionals may see the uterus and its structures with the use of medical imaging procedures including MRIs, hysteroscopies, and ultrasounds, which help with diagnosis and treatment planning.

The Uterus's Structure

Nestled between the bladder and the rectum in the pelvis, the uterus is a muscular, hollow structure. It is composed of three main layers: the serosa, which covers the uterus and acts as a protective barrier; the myometrium, which is composed of thick smooth muscle tissue and is responsible for the contractions of the uterus during labor and delivery; and the endometrium, which is the innermost layer and changes cyclically in response to hormone signals.

When not pregnant, the uterus has a pear-shaped form, but during pregnancy, it grows dramatically to accommodate the developing fetus. Its position and stability are preserved by the ligaments and muscles that support it within the pelvic cavity. The bottom portion of the uterus, known as the cervix, joins the vagina and acts as a birth canal when a woman gives birth as well as a conduit for the flow of menstrual blood.

Recognizing the anatomy of the uterus is crucial for the diagnosis and management of endometriosis, adenomyosis, and uterine fibroids, among other gynecological disorders. To guide patients' treatment decisions, medical experts evaluate the size, shape, and condition of the uterus and its layers using diagnostic methods like hysteroscopy, MRIs, and transvaginal ultrasounds.

The Endometrium's Function In The Menstrual Cycle

The endometrium, which is the deepest layer of the uterus, is subject to dynamic changes caused by hormones during the menstrual cycle. Its main purpose is to create an environment that is favorable for the implantation of embryos and the growth of fetuses throughout pregnancy. The endometrium sheds during menstruation, signaling the start of a new cycle, in the absence of pregnancy.

Under the influence of progesterone and estrogen, the endometrium thickens during the menstrual cycle in preparation for pregnancy. In the event of conception, the developing fetus is supported and grows when the embryo implants into the endometrial lining. In the absence of pregnancy, hormone levels drop, resulting in the endometrial lining shed and the onset of menstruation.

The responsiveness of the endometrium to hormone fluctuations is essential for reproductive health and conception. The endometrium can be affected by disorders such as endometriosis, polyps, and hyperplasia, which may necessitate medical intervention to restore normal menstrual periods and fertility.

Control Of Hormones

The menstrual cycle and the operation of the uterus are fundamentally influenced by hormonal regulation. The ovaries, pituitary gland, and hypothalamus work together to regulate hormone release that regulates endometrial lining growth, development, and shedding. During the first half of the menstrual cycle, estrogen, which is mostly produced by the ovaries, drives the growth and thickening of the endometrium.

In the second part of the menstrual cycle, progesterone, another hormone generated by the ovaries, works to further grow and prime the endometrium for potential pregnancy. Estrogen and progesterone levels fall in the absence of fertilization, indicating the endometrial lining's shedding and the start of menstruation.

Hormonal imbalances can result in irregular menstrual periods, infertility, and gynecological disorders such as hypothalamic amenorrhea or polycystic ovarian syndrome (PCOS). In certain situations, hormone treatment and medicine may be used to control hormone levels and return menstruation to normal.

Typical Uterine Conditions

The uterus can be impacted by several common illnesses, which can result in symptoms like irregular bleeding, pelvic pain, and infertility. Benign growths in the uterine muscle tissue known as uterine fibroids can strain on nearby organs and result in excessive menstrual flow. Endometriosis is a painful and infertile condition that arises when tissue resembling the lining of the uterus grows outside of it.

Adenomyosis is a disorder that causes pelvic pain and heavy periods because endometrial tissue develops into the uterus's muscular walls. Small growths called uterine polyps that are affixed to the uterine wall may also result in irregular bleeding and, if they become symptomatic, may require removal.

Healthcare professionals can see these conditions and choose the most effective course of treatment with the use of diagnostic instruments including MRIs, ultrasounds, and hysteroscopies. Treatment options may include hormone therapy, medicines, minimally invasive procedures like endometrial ablation, or surgical interventions like hysterectomy, depending on the patient's preferences and the severity of their symptoms.

Imaging Methods And Diagnostic Instruments

To assess uterine health and diagnose gynecological disorders, diagnostic instruments, and imaging methods are essential.

Transvaginal ultrasonography aids medical professionals in evaluating the size, shape, and health of the uterus and ovaries by producing images of these organs using high-frequency sound waves. Uterine fibroids, adenomyosis, and other anomalies can be diagnosed with the help of comprehensive images of the uterus and associated structures provided by magnetic resonance imaging, or MRI.

Doctors can use a thin, flexible tube with a light and camera attached to perform a minimally invasive technique called hysteroscopy, which allows them to look into the uterus.

By directly seeing the uterine cavity, it can be used for the diagnosis and treatment of fibroids, uterine polyps, and other structural disorders.

Healthcare professionals may accurately diagnose patients with uterine diseases and provide individualized treatment strategies for them thanks to these diagnostic tools and imaging procedures. Healthcare professionals can suggest the best interventions to enhance uterine health and general well-being by knowing the underlying causes of symptoms and anomalies.

CHAPTER TWO
CONTRAINDICATIONS AND INDICATIONS

For women who have not responded to conventional therapies, such as medication, endometrial ablation is a surgery used to manage heavy monthly bleeding. It is usually advised for women who are done having children or who do not intend to have children in the future. Anemia, exhaustion, and other symptoms caused by heavy monthly bleeding that severely impairs a woman's quality of life are the primary indications for endometrial ablation.

On the other hand, endometrial ablation might not be appropriate or useful in other situations. Women who still want children have contraindications because this surgery can seriously lower fertility or increase the risk of pregnancy. Additionally, women with active pelvic infections, precancerous diseases, or specific uterine anatomical anomalies should not use it.

Your healthcare practitioner will review your medical history and order any required tests before endometrial ablation to make sure you are a good candidate for the treatment. This assessment aids in locating any elements that might compromise the treatment's efficacy or endanger your health.

The Cause Of Excessive Menstrual Bleeding

Menorrhagia, or heavy menstrual bleeding, is a frequent issue that affects women and can have a major negative influence on everyday activities and quality of life. Menstrual periods that are unusually heavy, protracted, or both are its defining characteristics. Symptoms of this illness include bleeding that lasts longer than usual, soaking through pads or tampons quickly, and needing to use double protection.

By removing the endometrium, the lining of the uterus from which heavy menstrual bleeding originates, endometrial ablation seeks to minimize or completely stop the flow. When more conventional therapies, such as medication, have failed or are not appropriate for the patient, this surgery is taken into consideration.

Polyps, Fibroids, And Additional Growths

Benign growths in the uterus called fibroids and polyps can cause excessive menstrual bleeding. Polyps are tiny, non-cancerous growths that can form on the uterine lining, whereas fibroids are non-cancerous growths composed of muscle tissue. Inconsistent bleeding patterns, pelvic pain, and other symptoms may be brought on by these growths.

It's critical to determine whether fibroids, polyps, or other uterine structural anomalies exist before undergoing endometrial ablation. The success of the ablation operation may be impacted by these growths, contingent on their size, quantity, and position. To maximize the benefits of the ablation, they might occasionally need to be taken out or given different care.

Knowing What Endometrial Hyperplasia Is

The term "endometrial hyperplasia" describes the thickening of the endometrium, which lines the uterus. An imbalance in the hormones progesterone and estrogen, which control the menstrual cycle, may be the cause.

Atypical hyperplasia, a precancerous condition that raises the chance of developing uterine cancer, can occasionally arise from endometrial hyperplasia.

It's critical to rule out atypical or endometrial hyperplasia before conducting endometrial ablation. These ailments may necessitate additional testing or care and may have an impact on the procedure's suitability.

To determine the thickness and condition of the endometrium, your healthcare professional might suggest imaging testing or an endometrial biopsy.

Who Must Steer Clear Of Endometrial Ablation?

Not everyone can benefit from endometrial ablation, and there are a few signs that might suggest this isn't the best course of action for you.

Endometrial ablation can drastically lower fertility or increase the risk of pregnancy, thus women who still want children should avoid it. Women who have reached childbearing age or who do not intend to become pregnant in the future are the target audience for this operation.

Moreover, women who have ongoing pelvic infections, uterine cancer precancerous diseases, or other anatomical defects may not be good candidates for endometrial ablation.

If the ablation is carried out, these disorders may have an impact on the outcome or present health hazards.

Essential Pre-procedure Examinations

Several pre-procedure tests are usually carried out to determine your appropriateness for endometrial ablation and to guarantee your safety. These examinations could consist of:

Pelvic examination: To determine the dimensions, form, and state of your ovaries and uterus.

Ultrasonography: To view the uterus and identify any anomalies that could impact the surgery, such as fibroids, polyps, or other growths.

Endometrial Biopsy: This procedure involves taking a tiny sample of tissue from the endometrium, the lining that lines the uterus, to look for any anomalies, such as hyperplasia or malignant alterations.

Lab testing: To analyze your overall health, such as blood tests to determine your blood clotting function and to screen for anemia.

Pregnancy Test: To ensure that you are not expecting, as endometrial ablation is not advised for women who are expecting.

By using these tests, your healthcare practitioner can assess whether endometrial ablation is the right surgery for you and whether you need to undergo any extra treatments or take any precautions before it.

Comprehending the outcomes of these examinations guarantees that you have the safest and most efficient care for your ailment.

CHAPTER THREE
ENDOMETRIAL ABLATION PROCEDURE TYPES

Ablation Of Thermal Balloons

By dissolving the uterine lining, thermal balloon ablation is a minimally invasive surgery used to treat heavy menstrual bleeding. A balloon catheter is introduced into the uterus during this surgery by passing through the cervix. After that, the balloon is filled with a heated fluid—typically saline—that is cycled into the uterus for a predetermined amount of time. The fluid's heat effectively cauterizes the uterine lining, resulting in scarring and decreased bleeding over time.

Compared to standard surgery, this technique has the advantage of being able to be done as an outpatient treatment under local anesthesia or mild sedation, which shortens the recovery period. After thermal balloon ablation, the majority of women have a significant reduction in menstrual bleeding; many even achieve amenorrhea, no periods, or noticeably lighter periods.

Ablation Using Radiofrequency

Another treatment for severe menstrual bleeding is radiofrequency ablation or RF ablation. A thin, flexible device is placed into the uterus during this surgery by passing through the cervix. The endometrial tissue lining the uterus is destroyed by the radiofrequency energy the device releases, which also produces heat. The tissue is successfully cauterized by this heat, which lowers its propensity to cause menstrual bleeding.

Although local anesthetic may be utilized, radiofrequency ablation is usually done in an outpatient setting and does not require general anesthesia. Many women recover quickly, returning to their regular activities in a day or two. It is especially appropriate for ladies who want to stay away from more intrusive surgical procedures or hormonal therapies.

Ablation Via Hydrothermal Process

Heavy menstrual bleeding can be treated using a technique called hydrothermal ablation, or HTA, which involves heating saline solution.

A specifically made tool is put into the uterus through the cervix during this surgery. The endometrial tissue is successfully destroyed by the hot saline that is released by the device and circulates throughout the uterus.

This approach has the benefit of being minimally invasive and frequently being done as an outpatient surgery.

Most women can resume their regular activities in a matter of days, and it is usually well tolerated and requires little recovery time. Women who want to keep their uterus intact and choose a non-hormonal treatment option should consider hydrothermal ablation.

Ablation Of Microwaves

One relatively newer method for endometrial ablation is microwave ablation. A tiny probe is sent through the cervix and into the uterus during this operation. The endometrial tissue lining the uterus is heated and destroyed by the microwave energy released by the probe. In many cases, this damage leads to a decrease in monthly flow or even amenorrhea.

General anesthesia is not necessary for microwave ablation procedures, which are usually done as outpatient procedures. Most women recover quickly, returning to their regular activities in a day or two. For women who want to cure severe menstrual bleeding quickly and effectively without using hormones, this procedure is beneficial.

Freezing

The process of cryoablation involves destroying the uterine endometrial lining with extremely cold temperatures. A probe is placed into the uterus through the cervix during this operation. The endometrial tissue is subsequently frozen and destroyed when the probe cools to an extremely low temperature. The tissue cannot regrow as a result of this destruction, which lessens menstrual bleeding.

Although local anesthetic may be utilized, general anesthesia is not normally necessary for cryoablation, which is done as an outpatient treatment. Many women recover quickly enough to return to their regular activities in a matter of days. Women who want to avoid more invasive surgical procedures and prefer a non-hormonal treatment alternative will find this method especially beneficial.

38

CHAPTER FOUR

BEFORE THE PROCEDURE

It is imperative to make proper preparations before endometrial ablation to guarantee a seamless treatment and speedy recovery. Usually, your doctor will walk you through a series of measures to make sure you're mentally and physically prepared.

Preliminary Medical Assessment

Your healthcare physician does a comprehensive medical evaluation at the start of the process. Your medical history, present menstrual bleeding symptoms, and any prior therapies you may have received are all discussed during this evaluation.

It's critical to reveal any allergies or medical issues you may have, along with any drugs you use at the moment.

The medical staff can evaluate your general health and decide whether endometrial ablation is a good option for you with the use of this information.

Pre-Procedure Drugs And Their Applications

Your doctor may prescribe medicine to get your uterus ready for the treatment, depending on your particular situation.

These drugs may consist of hormone therapies or substances that thin the uterine lining, improving the efficiency of the ablation procedure. Improving results and creating the ideal atmosphere for the process are the main objectives.

Dietary Guidelines And Restrictions

You may receive dietary instructions from your doctor to follow in the days before your surgery. Usually, these recommendations entail abstaining from particular foods or drinks that can have an impact on the surgery or recuperation.

To reduce risks and guarantee the greatest outcomes from the ablation, it is imperative that you strictly adhere to these directions.

Getting Ready For Procedure Day

There are a few doable things you may do to physically prepare yourself as the operation day draws near.

This includes making plans for getting to and from the medical institution, making sure you have clothes that fit well, and bringing any supplies your doctor prescribes.

It's crucial to schedule any time off from work or other commitments to allow for enough rest and recuperation following the surgery.

Emotional And Psychological Readiness

Having any kind of medical treatment done can be very emotionally taxing. Feeling apprehensive or uneasy about the impending ablation is common. It can be beneficial to discuss your sentiments and concerns with your healthcare professional.

They can answer any questions you may have and give you information about what to expect throughout the treatment. Before the surgery, practicing relaxation techniques like deep breathing or meditation might also help you feel less anxious.

CHAPTER FIVE

DAY OF THE PROCEDURE

You've been waiting anxiously for this day: the endometrial ablation operation. The goal of this outpatient surgery is to remove or destroy the uterine endometrial lining to decrease or cease monthly flow.

You will likely arrive at the surgical center early in the day, so make arrangements for a companion to provide support and help when you get there.

Process Of Arrival And Check-In

When you arrive, the surgery center's welcoming personnel will greet you. They will assist you with the check-in process, which entails confirming your medical history, and personal information, and understanding the specifics of the operation.

It might be necessary for you to take off any jewelry and accessories and change into a hospital gown.

Options For Anesthesia And Their Impacts

You and your healthcare team will talk about anesthesia alternatives before the process starts. The particular procedure that is planned, your preferences, and your medical history will all play a role in the sort of anesthesia that is utilized.

There are two possible options: general anesthesia, which would render you unconscious during the treatment, or local anesthetic, which will simply numb the area surrounding your uterus.

Every anesthetic kind has implications and things to think about. During the process, you can stay awake and conscious with minimal discomfort thanks to local anesthesia.

Conversely, a temporary state of unconsciousness brought on by general anesthetic guarantees that you are oblivious to the process. Your medical team will walk you through the advantages and disadvantages of each option so you can make an educated choice.

Overview Of The Process Step-By-Step

After the anesthesia is given and you're ready, the process will start. To view the cervix, your doctor will first introduce a speculum into your vagina. After that, a thin device known as a hysteroscope will be carefully inserted into the uterus through the cervix. With the camera built into this hysteroscope, your doctor can view your uterus while keeping an eye on the process on a screen.

The endometrial lining will then be removed or destroyed using specialized instruments. While there are many different ways to accomplish the same goal, common approaches include using heat, cold, microwave, or radiofrequency energy. To achieve complete therapy while avoiding injury to adjacent tissues, your doctor will carefully maneuver the equipment.

Length And Experience In The Rehab Room

Depending on the approach selected and the complexity of your case, the operation can take anywhere from 15 minutes to an hour. Following the treatment, you'll be sent to a recovery room where medical staff will keep an eye on your vital signs and make sure you're comfortable while the anesthesia wears off.

Quick Postoperative Care

During the first few hours after your endometrial ablation, you could feel a little uncomfortable and have cramps. These are common symptoms that can be controlled with painkillers that your doctor has recommended.

To give your body time to heal, it's crucial to take it easy and stay away from physically demanding activities for the remainder of the day.

Specific post-procedure instructions, such as when you can resume regular activities, showering, and food, will be given by your healthcare team.

Additionally, they will arrange a follow-up meeting to assess your progress and address any worries or inquiries you might have.

Recall that each woman's experience with endometrial ablation is unique, so don't be afraid to let your doctor know if you are uncomfortable or experiencing any strange symptoms.

CHAPTER SIX

RESTORATION AFTER PROCEDURE

The initial post-procedure recovery phase following endometrial ablation is critical for maximizing healing and minimizing discomfort. Before being sent home, you might need to spend a brief amount of time in the recovery room while your status is monitored. Although everyone's recovery process is unique, there are some general rules to abide by to speed up healing and minimize any potential issues.

For a few days following the treatment, minor discomfort that resembles menstruation cramps is not uncommon.

To relieve this pain, your doctor might recommend using painkillers. For your body to fully recover from the initial period of recuperation, you must rest and refrain from physically demanding activities.

Watery or bloody vaginal discharge is another common symptom experienced by some women. The tissue that was treated during the ablation is being lost by your body, which is why this discharge is normal. Tampons should not be used at this time; instead, sanitary pads should be used to lower the risk of infection.

It's critical to abide by your doctor's advice about dosage, activity level, and any special care requirements. If you have any questions or notice any strange symptoms while recovering, don't be afraid to ask your healthcare professional for advice.

Normal Timetable For Recuperation

After endometrial ablation, recovery times can vary, but most patients are back to their regular routines in a few days to a week.

Initially, you might have mild to severe pelvic pain and cramps, which can be treated with over-the-counter painkillers or prescription drugs.

It's best to rest and stay away from heavy lifting and intense activity during the first 24 to 48 hours following the surgery.

Walking and other light exercises are recommended to improve circulation and facilitate healing. Vaginal discharge is possible, but it should progressively go away in the first several weeks.

Many women report feeling much better by the end of the first week, at which point they can resume their regular activities and work.

You must keep an eye on your symptoms and follow your doctor's recommendations on any activity limitations.

Although recovery times could vary, most people recover fully in 1 to 2 weeks. You must show up for any follow-up appointments you have with your doctor during this time so they can evaluate your healing process and answer any questions you may have.

Handling Soreness And Unease

An essential part of your recovery after endometrial ablation is managing your pain and discomfort. You can get cramps just after the surgery that resemble menstruation cramps.

To ease this discomfort, your healthcare professional might suggest over-the-counter remedies or prescribe painkillers.

Taking warm baths or placing a heating pad on your stomach might also help reduce cramps. You can lessen discomfort even more by finding a comfortable resting posture that supports your legs and back enough.

Get in touch with your healthcare practitioner for a more thorough assessment if you suffer from severe or ongoing pain that does not go away with medication or other treatments. It's critical to take care of pain as soon as possible to maintain your comfort and well-being as you heal.

Activity Limitations And Suggestions

It's critical to adhere to certain activity limits after endometrial ablation to encourage appropriate healing and lower the chance of problems.

Steer clear of demanding exercises, hard lifting, and strenuous activities in the initial days following the surgery.

Walking and other light exercises are recommended to improve circulation and speed healing. Adapt your exercise level to your feelings and gradually raise it, but pay attention to your body and refrain from overexerting yourself.

After the treatment, most women can return to their regular activities within a week; however, it is crucial to refrain from any activities that can put strain on the pelvic area or create discomfort.

Depending on the type of ablation treatment used and your particular situation, your healthcare professional will provide you with precise guidelines.

Do not hesitate to ask your doctor for specific advice if you have any questions or concerns regarding what activities are safe to engage in while recovering.

Indications Of Complications And When To Consult A Physician

Even though endometrial ablation is usually regarded as safe, it's crucial to be informed of any possible issues that can occur during the healing process. Please get in touch with your physician right once if you encounter any of the following symptoms:

Prolonged or intense vaginal bleeding that goes beyond what is regarded as typical following surgery.

severe stomach ache for which there is no treatment with painkillers.

chills or fever, which could be signs of an infection.

discharge from the vagina that smells bad or symptoms of an infection.

considerable pain when urinating or difficulty urinating.

These signs may point to complications including infection, uterine perforation, or other problems that need to be treated right once. Prompt action can guarantee a smooth healing process and help stop additional issues.

Recheck Schedules And Extended-Term Care

After endometrial ablation, follow-up visits are a crucial component of your long-term care and recuperation.

These consultations will be planned by your healthcare professional to track your healing process and answer any worries you may have.

Your doctor may do pelvic exams or ultrasound scans during follow-up appointments to evaluate the outcome of the ablation surgery and make sure your symptoms are getting better.

In addition, they will talk about any modifications to menstrual bleeding patterns and, if necessary, offer advice for contraception.

Monitoring your menstrual cycles and any changes in symptoms over time are part of long-term treatment. Even though many women can completely stop or drastically reduce their menstrual flow after endometrial ablation, maintaining general reproductive health requires regular gynecological exams.

Your unique needs and preferences may lead your doctor to suggest additional therapies or interventions.

Maintaining open lines of contact with your healthcare practitioner is essential to making sure you get the assistance and attention required for a full recovery and continued well-being.

CHAPTER SEVEN

OVERSIGHTING GOALS AND RESULTS

For individuals thinking about endometrial ablation, controlling expectations and comprehending the results are essential.

Reducing or eliminating monthly bleeding is usually the main objective of endometrial ablation. Individual results may vary, even though many women report a considerable decrease in menstrual flow or even the cessation of periods.

Results can be influenced by a variety of factors, including the type of ablation surgery used, the underlying reason for severe bleeding, and individual differences in responsiveness to treatment.

After recovering from the operation, patients can often anticipate a decrease in menstrual bleeding. While some people may experience lighter periods right once, others may experience improvements over several months.

It's crucial to set reasonable expectations and realize that while most women see a favorable difference, not everyone will have a total stop of their periods.

Anticipated Shifts In The Menstrual Cycle

Women frequently suffer alterations in their menstrual cycle after endometrial ablation. The most frequent result is a notable decrease in menstrual bleeding. Some women may experience very little or nonexistent menstruation.

Others may experience unpredictable or erratic times. It's crucial to remember that these modifications are typical reactions to the surgery and typically signify that severe menstrual bleeding has been successfully treated.

Following the treatment, patients should anticipate some initial soreness or cramping, which usually goes away in a few days. As the uterus heals, it's also typical to have a clear or watery vaginal discharge. These alterations typically go away on their own without assistance and are a normal part of the healing process.

Possible Issues And How To Handle Them

Endometrial ablation poses potential dangers, like any medical surgery, even if it is generally safe. Infection, hemorrhage, harm to adjacent organs, and the likelihood that the surgery won't produce the expected results are examples of potential consequences. Before opting to have the surgery, patients should be fully informed about these risks and have a thorough discussion with their healthcare physician.

Although they are uncommon, infections can happen after endometrial ablation. Fever, intensifying pelvic pain, or atypical discharge are indicators of infection.

Patients should get in touch with their healthcare professional right away for an assessment and treatment if any of these symptoms appear.

Benefits Over Time And Success Rates

For most patients, one of the long-term benefits of endometrial ablation is a considerable reduction in or removal of excessive monthly bleeding. Research indicates that a considerable number of women report long-lasting relief from their menstrual issues following the operation. This may result in increased vitality, a higher quality of life, and a decreased need for period hygiene products.

Success rates differ based on the kind of ablation technique used as well as personal characteristics like age and underlying medical issues. Overall, there is a high success rate in reducing menstrual bleeding, and the majority of women express satisfaction with the treatment's outcomes.

Effects On Pregnancy And Fertility

For women who hope to get pregnant in the future, endometrial ablation is not advised because it drastically lowers the likelihood of conceiving spontaneously.

Preterm birth, aberrant placental attachment, and miscarriage are among the issues that are more likely to occur in a pregnancy that results from ablation.

It's crucial for women thinking about ablation to talk to their doctor about their reproductive objectives and, if they want to become pregnant in the future, look into other options.

Case Studies And Patient Testimonials

Numerous women who have had endometrial ablation attest to favorable outcomes and notable enhancements in their standard of living. Testimonials from patients frequently highlight improved confidence in social and professional contexts, alleviation from symptoms like anemia and exhaustion, and decreased monthly flow. Case studies also show how well the process works to reduce severe menstrual bleeding and enhance general health.

For women thinking about endometrial ablation, these testimonies and case studies can offer insightful information that will help them make well-informed decisions on their medical alternatives. It's crucial to speak with a licensed healthcare professional to find out if endometrial ablation is the best option for your needs given your unique medical circumstances and treatment objectives.

CHAPTER EIGHT

COMMON QUESTIONS AND ANSWERS

The goal of endometrial ablation is to remove or destroy the uterine lining to lessen or stop severe monthly flow.

It's reasonable to have doubts and concerns considering its nature. These are a few typical questions:

Is ablation of the endometrium safe?

Indeed, endometrial ablation is usually regarded as safe when carried out by a qualified medical professional. As with any medical operation, there are risks associated with it, too, such as bleeding, infection, and anesthesia-related issues.

After the surgery, would my periods continue to occur?

After endometrial ablation, many women report noticeably lower periods or no periods at all. Some, though, can still experience minor bleeding or spotting, particularly in the months right after the surgery.

Does the process hurt during it?

Since the ablation is usually done under anesthetic, you shouldn't experience any pain during the process. Cramps and soreness following surgery are typical, although they can typically be controlled with painkillers.

Can endometrial ablation prevent me from becoming pregnant?

Birth control is not provided via endometrial ablation, and pregnancy is still possible. Pregnancies following the operation, however, are frequently high-risk and may result in problems. If you are of childbearing age, it is highly advised that you use effective contraception.

Tips For Comfort And Pain Management

In the Process

Under general, regional, or local anesthetic, the majority of endometrial ablation treatments are carried out. Taking into account the particulars of the treatment as well as your medical history, your doctor will talk you through the best option. Although there may be some slight discomfort, pain is typically effectively managed.

Postoperative Pain Management

Similar to menstruation cramps, post-procedure cramping is typical. Acetaminophen or ibuprofen, two over-the-counter pain relievers, can help reduce this discomfort. If required, your doctor might also recommend more potent painkillers.

Comfort Tips for Your Home

You can relieve cramps by placing a warm pad on your lower abdomen. Comfort and recuperation can also be enhanced by resting and avoiding heavy activity for a few days following the treatment. A healthy diet and enough water will aid in your body's general healing process.

Recuperation Period And Resume Of Regular Activities

The first phase of recovery

After the surgery, most women can return home a few hours later. For a few days to a few weeks, it's common to have some cramping, minor pain, and a watery or bloody discharge. It is recommended that you take this initial period to rest at home and avoid heavy lifting or intense activity.

Going Back to Our Regular Activities

In most cases, you can resume your regular activities and job in a few days. Pay attention to your body; if you're tired or uncomfortable, take it easy. Reintroduce physical activity gradually, and before starting up an exercise regimen or doing any heavy lifting again, see your doctor.

Aftercare

A few weeks following the operation, your healthcare professional will usually schedule a follow-up consultation to discuss any concerns and make sure the healing process is going well. Notify your doctor right away if you experience any unusual symptoms, such as intense pain, heavy bleeding, or infection symptoms (fever, foul-smelling discharge).

Pregnancy Risks and Fertility Issues

Effect on the Rate of Fertility

Because endometrial ablation destroys the uterine lining required for implantation, it greatly lowers the chance of becoming pregnant. It is not, however, a method of contraception. See your doctor about long-term birth control choices if you want to avoid getting pregnant.

Pregnancy Risks Following Ablation

Although uncommon, pregnancy following endometrial ablation carries potential risks for the fetus and the mother. It's possible for the uterine lining to fail during pregnancy, which could result in an ectopic pregnancy, miscarriage, or other issues. Utilize dependable contraception to prevent unplanned pregnancies.

Talks About Family Planning

Endometrial ablation might not be the ideal choice for you if you are thinking about getting pregnant in the future. With your healthcare practitioner, talk over your family planning objectives and look into nonreproductive alternatives for severe menstrual bleeding.

Expense, Coverage, And Grant Support

Recognizing the Expenses

The type of surgery, the fees charged by the healthcare practitioner, and the location of the procedure can all have a significant impact on the cost of endometrial ablation. The price might range from a few thousand to several thousand dollars on average.

Protection From Insurance

Endometrial ablation is often covered by insurance companies if it is considered medically necessary. To learn more about your coverage, including any potential out-of-pocket expenses, co-pays, or deductibles, contact your insurance provider.

Options for Financial Assistance

If you're worried about the expense, talk to your healthcare physician or the hospital's billing department about financial aid programs or payment arrangements. Certain institutions have resources to assist with the cost of the procedure, or they offer sliding scale pricing based on income.

Following Ablation, Long-Term Health And Wellness

Keeping an Eye on Your Health

It's crucial to schedule routine follow-up visits with your doctor to keep an eye on your recovery from an ablation. Any unexpected or persistent symptoms, such as extreme pain, copious bleeding, or infection symptoms, should be reported right away.

Modifications to Lifestyle

Maintaining a healthy lifestyle can help you stay well into the future. This entails eating a healthy, balanced diet, getting regular exercise, controlling stress, and quitting smoking. These actions can enhance your general well-being and possibly lessen the likelihood that your symptoms will reappear.

Emotional and Mental Wellbeing

Improving your mental and emotional health can result from respite from severe menstrual flow. Take part in relaxing activities and, if necessary, ask friends, family, or support groups for assistance.

Frequent Obstetrical Care

Follow your doctor's advice and keep up with routine gynecological checkups and screenings, such as Pap smears and pelvic exams. These are crucial for preserving reproductive health and identifying any possible problems early on.

www.ingramcontent.com/pod-product-compliance
Lightning Source LLC
Chambersburg PA
CBHW071842210526
45479CB00001B/253